Kate's A-Z Of Healing:

From one Survivor Heart to Another

I0117221

Kate Swift

chipmunkapublishing
the mental health publisher

Published by
Chipmunkapublishing
PO Box 6872
Brentwood
Essex CM13 1ZT
United Kingdom

http://www.chipmunkapublishing.com

Edited by Fran Harvey

ISBN   978-1-84991-877-0

Chipmunkapublishing   gratefully   acknowledge   the support of Arts Council England.

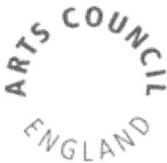

Dedication
This book is dedicated to my inner child and to yours.
This book is a fulfilment of a promise I made to her that I
would help others to never feel as alone as she once
did. I hope through the pages of this book you will hear
her voice, the one which is saying "We are healing...and
you can too"

Kate Swift

Introduction

This book began as a personal challenge to complete an alphabetical list based on healing. As I worked my way through the alphabet, I realised how 'key' many of the things I have listed were to my own healing journey (a journey which is ongoing). I shared a few pages with our peer to peer support group and they were well received... One member said the contents so resonated with her that she had goose bumps whilst reading. I came to realise how helpful my list may be for survivors everywhere. There are many excellent books on healing written by professionals. This book is different... this book has been written by a survivor of C.S.A for other survivors of C.S.A. It is not by any means a substantial read in volume however I believe the contents might have a substantial impact on the reader. This is intended to be one of those books which you can dip in and out of at your own leisure. You may need to read & re-read some of the pages several times over. I hope this book will help to inspire you on your own A-Z of healing. All the Photographic letters throughout the book are my own work too. Creativity and photography are wonderful tools in my own healing. This book is no substitute for professional help and advice, think of it as a 'starter' or a 'dessert' with professional help being the main course. I have no formal training in this field other than the school of life which comes from living with CSA from the age of 8 through to 16 and the aftermath since. I have been living and learning the contents of what is now this book. I hope this book will give you insight and strength for your own journey.

Kate Swift

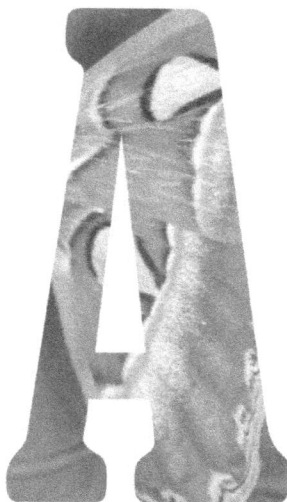

Is for... Allowing

'A' is for allowing... Allowing yourself to feel, to be, to mend, to be cared about, to take the time you need. Allowing yourself the same care and compassion you show to others. Allowing yourself the same respect and esteem that you give to others. We need to allow ourselves to feel broken (a brave thing to do) so that we can begin to mend, rather than pretending to the world (maybe even to yourself) that you are 'fine' when inside you're crumbling. We need to allow the right people to help us rather than feeling like we did as a child that we have to manage alone. Most importantly of all allow yourself to be the best 'you' that you can be. Refuse to let your past steal away your future.

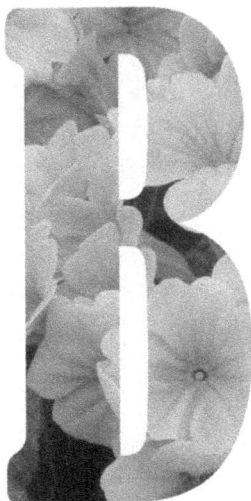

Is for... Banishing

'B' is for banishing... Banishing the blame and the guilt many survivors feel following on from abuse. Learning through therapeutic work that it was never our shame and guilt to carry or own. Learning to throw it back to the abuser where it rightfully belongs. Banishing the negative voices in your head which tell you that you are not good enough... these are untruths. When we begin to banish the negatives, they can be replaced with healthier thought patterns. As someone who has been through CSA you may be left with so many messages and responsibilities that were never yours to own. To banish something or someone is to forbid them from being around you... is it time to work on banishing things from your life which have hurt you?

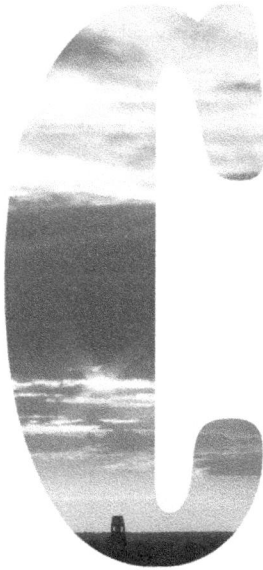

Is for... Creating

'C' is for creating.... You can create the future that you want for yourself; you can create new hopes and new possibilities. You can create an environment around you with the people who build you up, not those who are waiting to knock you down. You can't change your yesterdays but you can start creating your tomorrows. Begin creating opportunities for you to be happy. Be aware of the people in your life, how they treat you and why... don't allow others to treat you badly. You deserve to be treated with love and respect. Tomorrow is a blank canvas and the canvas is yours to create anything you want to on it... what will you create?

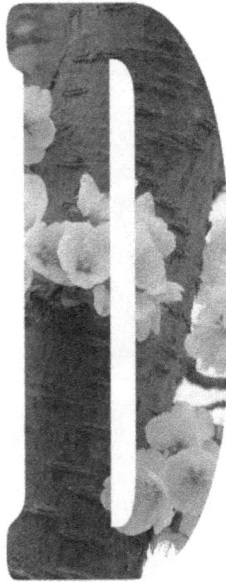

Is for... Dream

'D' is for dream... Dare to dream for 'you'. Dreams can come in any size... even if something feels too big to achieve... it doesn't make it a fact! Build your dreams and don't allow anyone to take them from you. I received a birthday card quite a few years ago now and I've never forgotten what it said... 'Follow your dreams and your heart will always be happy'. Even just feeling happy can feel like an impossible dream... your life can be so much better than you dare to believe... just keep on keeping on!

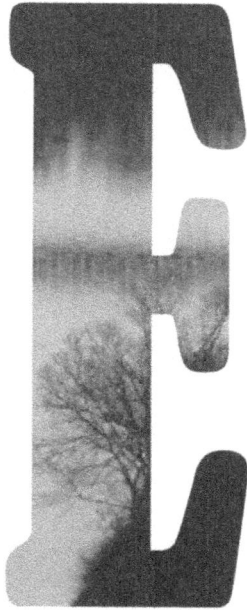

Is for... Express

'E' is for Express... how you feel. Find safe ways to be able to let go of your negative emotions. We keep so much bottled up inside of ourselves and if we can learn to face it (with the right support) ...then we can begin to let it go. Expressing how you feel doesn't always have to be about telling another person... you could write, draw, paint, sing... whatever helps you to let the negative feelings go away safely.

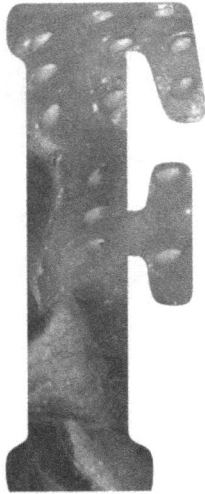

Is for... Flourish

'F' is for Flourish... you and I have not been born merely to survive; we were not born to know only what we have had to endure so far. You were born to flourish and to experience joy. Here to grow from the deep, dark ground and to blossom into beauty... Look for opportunities to be the person you want to be and know that you are just as entitled as the next person to be happy... to be able to flourish. Be with the people in your life who build you up, not knock you down. Spend time doing the things that make you feel happy and contented. If you want something to flourish you have to treat it well and take care of it... you deserve to be treated well and taken care of.

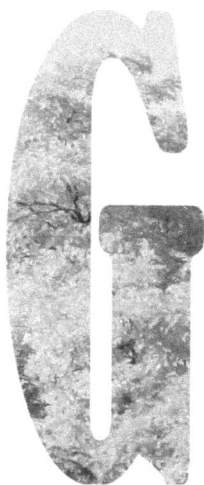

Is for... Grieve

'G' is for Grieving... in the process of healing and being able to move forwards survivors have some grieving to do. We need to grieve for the loss of childhood, or maybe the parenting that we never experienced, maybe for the loss of our innocence. These are all BIG things which every child deserves to have... a safe, loving, nurturing environment. It is okay/natural to feel sad about these things. It is a part of the healing journey. Allow yourself time to stand still and grieve what you lost, grieve what you never had and should have had. Because once you have spent some time 'feeling' it, the power of the grief can begin to diffuse and you can begin to move forward. Freed up to enjoy what you have now and what shapes your future.

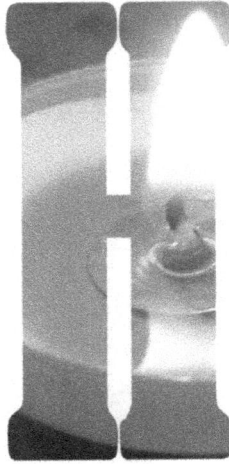

Is for... Help

'H' is for Help... at some point everyone needs help and asking for help is not a sign of weakness. Recognising that you need help and asking for it is good self care. Help comes in many different forms... what is right for one person, may not work for another. In getting therapeutic help I saw several counsellors/therapists before settling with one who I felt really cared & could really help me... and he did. Often a survivor tells me they asked for help in the past and either did not receive it or it wasn't right for them. It's tempting to want to throw in the towel at that point but it is so important to keep going. You 'DESERVE' help and although it may not come easily please persist in getting what you need & deserve.

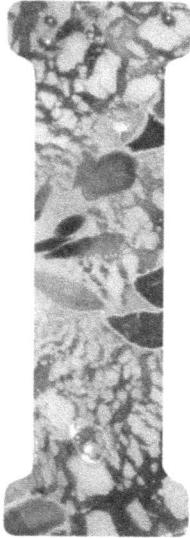

Is For... Instinct

'I' is for Instinct... I have a strong and very accurate gut instinct. I have heard lots of survivors say the same thing. Learning to listen to our gut instinct... learning to take action and follow that instinct is a positive thing. I can recall a few occasions in recent years where my gut instinct was telling me something... I decided to go the other way and just hoped it would work out fine... I was wrong and I learnt that the hard way. More and more I am learning to follow that inborn impulse... it seems to want to look out for me and that can only be for my good.

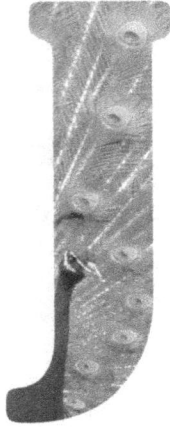

Is for... Justice

'J' is for Justice... Justice is a very emotive word in our world, where we have been violated so badly. More Survivors don't ever get justice through a legal system than those who do. My abuser received a 'police caution'... no justice in that I feel. So I went on to make my own personal justice... by opting to live the best, the most fulfilling and happiest life I can lead. By taking back the power and refusing to allow him to continue having a daily negative reign over my life. Of course this didn't come easy or happen overnight but slowly and surely I have my own personal justice. Now to quote the lyrics of a Kelly Clarkson song... 'What doesn't kill you makes you stronger' ...I am indeed stronger and justice will be mine because my life is mine... I took it back.

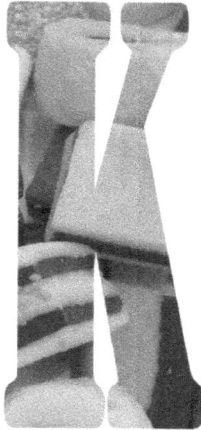

Is for... Kaleidoscope

'K' is for Kaleidoscope... I often think that life is like looking through a Kaleidoscope... one day it seems this way, another day you look and it seems totally different. One day life is looking beautiful another day – another twist of the Kaleidoscope and you may not like what you are seeing. Try to remember that if the picture of your life right now is not what you want... further down the line the tide will turn, the pieces of the kaleidoscope will fall into different places... and things will look more hopeful, brighter, more how you want them to be. Difficult days have not come to stay although when you are in the middle of them it can feel like forever. Consider them pieces in life's Kaleidoscope of colours and patterns... ever-changing and often for the better.

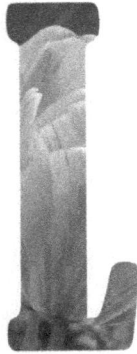

Is for... Like

'L' is for Like... So many Survivors are left with such a low or even no self-esteem and sense of self. We spend so long living in the shadows of blame or shame. When we can accept the truth of who we are... the –truth- and not the lies that our past feeds into us; the kind of lies which whisper into our very core that we are rubbish, unworthy, no good, unlovable etc. When the truth of the matter is that we are 'Survivors'... we survived some of the worst crimes that one can do to another person. We are blameless... we were not responsible for what happened to us... We were children, trying to make sense of something which adults often fail to understand. Learning to like yourself may take you a long time and a lot of work (as it did me) but it is such a key part of our healing. I had to make an epic journey inside of myself from hate to self acceptance. My wish would be that every survivor can fulfil that journey within themselves.

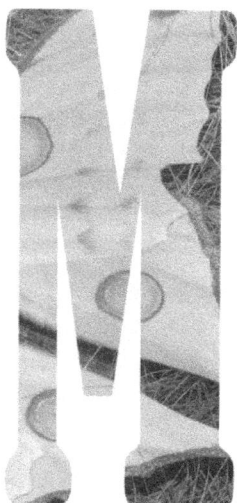

Is for... Mosaic

'M' is for Mosaic... Beautiful works of art are made from little pieces. I can remember the times when I felt my life was in little pieces and I didn't know how to gather them together... or even if it was possible. That is why in this instance M is for Mosaic because if you feel like your life is in bits, I want you to know that something new and wonderful can be created. Piece by piece you can shape your life into how you want it to be. You are the master crafter of your own soul, use the tools available to you and create something new. If you don't like where you are now either inwardly or geographically, begin to work on changing the direction of your life... piece by piece you can achieve it.

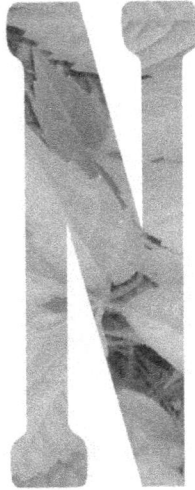

Is for...

'N' is for Nurture... This one I believe to be quite a challenge for many survivors. When I learnt to accept & embrace my inner child, I felt more whole and more healed as an adult person. It was quite some journey because it began with me feeling nothing but hatred for her. With time and work I came to realise that she was not the bad person in all of this. In fact my inner child was innocent - blameless. From that point onwards I tried to nurture her rather than as I had in the past ignore her. Instead of silencing her plea for attention, I allowed her to have a voice through my writing, artwork or by doing something that she would like to do. I quickly learnt that when the child inside of me felt nurtured and safe... the adult felt the same way. Instead of fighting with that part of myself, I made peace with it... with her. As a child I could not do anything to protect myself or to stop what was happening. As an adult I can protect my inner child and I can ensure to the best of my ability that she comes to no more harm. I can meet her un-met needs and just like a small child who is repeatedly asking for something... when the need is met they are quiet.

When I spent time nurturing my inner child she stopped invading my life with sad and painful thoughts. Now I like to look after her and in doing so I am looking after myself.

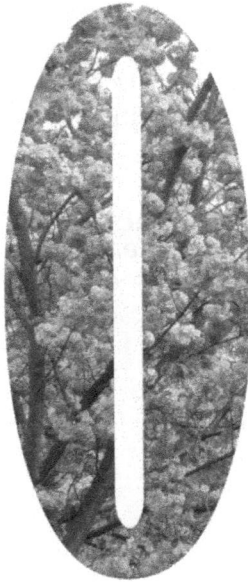

Is for...

'O' is for Ongoing... I believe the journey to healing is something that will be ongoing for me. I am so much better than I was and I hope to be better than I am now in the future. I get a lot of encouragement from looking back just long enough to see how far I have come. It gives me hope that the future will indeed be far brighter than my past. Every new day that breaks is an opportunity to heal some more, to learn something new, to be more of the person you want to be. Look how far you have come in your own journey, and then just imagine how far you can go... and smile.

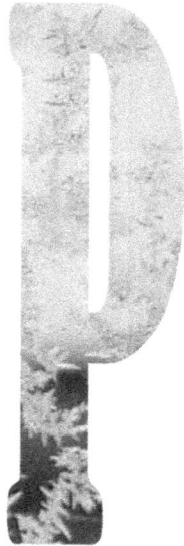

Is for...

'P' is for Pace... Healing is not a race and it is such an individual thing. We often compare ourselves to those around us. I have often had a survivor say to me that their abuse was only on a few occasions or that it was much more insignificant than other stories they read about. I always say that if you were abused, there is no measuring stick... if you were abused once or many times over... it affected you and you deserve help and support. In the same way we can feel frustrated that we are not 'mended' yet... & compare ourselves to others who may seem to be so much further down the healing road. We all had to start from somewhere and that starting point is different for each person. Progress can seem so slow and insignificant, especially when you are in great emotional pain. We need to learn to pace ourselves and to go at our own speed. You cannot rush the healing process. Therapy will take as long as it is going to take for each person.

I remember I used to think that I 'should' be better by now and I often said it in therapy. I have always remembered my Psychologists response: Think about the length of time (years) the damage was done to you... then you realise it cannot be fixed in a short space of time. So long as you keep going in the right direction and you have the help you need... you will get to wherever it is you need to be... pace yourself.

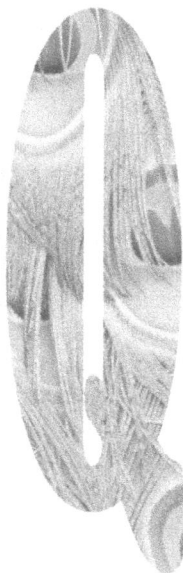

Is for...

'Q' is for Question... We often assume that Doctors, Therapists etc know what is best for us. I would like to think that in the vast majority they do, however it is okay to question people. If you are not sure about your treatment or something being suggested for you... question it... say what you need to say. This is –your-healing journey, if you are unsure about something or you feel something really isn't right for you speak up about it. Sometimes we do know what is best for ourselves and when something really isn't right for us. Equally you may know that you could really benefit from a treatment or a talking therapy which you're not getting... again I would say question it, talk to the people helping you. On this journey there is someone else who we probably need to question... ourselves. We need to question all those negative self beliefs we may have grown up adopting as our own framework. The spoken and often unspoken messages that we receive as a result of abuse... messages such as "You are worthless" which can play on a loop system in our very core self. These need to be called into question as we explore what happened to us and we look towards healing.

These negative self beliefs were given to us to make someone else feel better than us; feel more powerful than us, maintain some control perhaps. This is not who you are... those are labels... labels are for boxes and not for people I like to say. You need to question yourself and discover firstly who you are not then you can begin to learn to love and respect the person you are. As you do this some real concrete healing can take place and your self esteem will begin to lift.

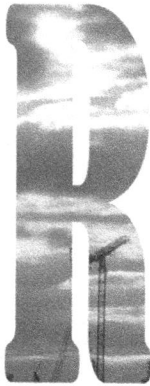

Is for...

'R' is for Refuel... Our emotions are like a fuel tank and many of us tend to be people who 'give'. We might give our time, our energy, our support to one thing or another. What we need to remember is that if we constantly are giving out or being emotionally drained... we need our emotional tank refuelled. We need to create leisure time, relaxing time, the opportunity for laughter, time with people who make you feel good etc. All of these things re-stock our emotional fuel tank so that we can give out and not be running on empty ourselves. The healing journey through childhood sexual abuse is immensely draining and therefore self care is so important. We need to make the time and create the opportunities to have positive experiences which give us positive emotions. Nobody can run on empty indefinitely... do you need to refuel your emotional tank right now?

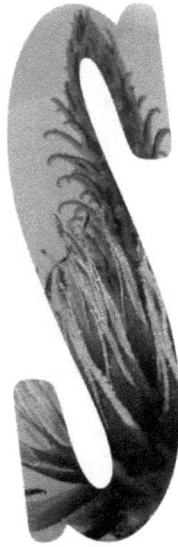

Is for...

'S' is for Survivor... Firstly I know I was a victim of C.S.A and for several years once it had stopped I still felt like a victim. Why... because it invaded my life every single day, not a day went by when I didn't think about some aspect of it. However we can go on from victim to survivor. I will always have been a victim of this crime; however I choose to be a survivor. I spent several years feeling like I was 'existing' rather than living the life I wanted to live, more so that the life I had wanted was no longer obtainable for me. As a victim I was injured... the crime committed against me made me suffer, not just at the time but left a legacy. After a lot of help and a lot of work on myself, I began to feel less like the 'victim'. My life started to be re-shaped into something far more positive and purposeful. That is why I believe 'S' is for Survivor... we have (thank goodness) survived what happened to us in our early life. As powerless children our abuser could take and maintain control... as adults we can take back that power. As adults we can change the landscape by working our way through the things which hold us back.

I would far rather consider myself a survivor than a victim of C.S.A. For me it is far more hopeful and empowering to know I survived in spite of once being a victim... I am a survivor and I also intend to go one further than that and thrive!

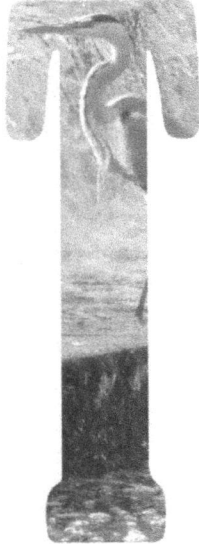

Is for...

'T' is for Thrive... Following on from surviving my aim is also to 'thrive'. The days of feeling like I was existing rather than truly living once seemed endless... I don't want to just exist... I don't want to just survive... I want to learn how to thrive. To thrive is to live life richly (not in a material sense) but to be happy and healthy. Building a healthy life that on the whole makes you feel balanced and positive is thriving. Spending time investing in your own well being is time invested in learning how to thrive... how to live beyond existing and even beyond surviving. Who you are and what you want your life to be needs to be tended to like a gardener nurtures a garden. It can take a lot of work to have a beautiful garden... but when it blooms and flourishes you see the work you put in bearing fruit. I believe the same is true of the work you put into yourself. After CSA we are left with a heap of internal (and external) mess to clear up. We need to work our way through the wasteland, clearing the rubbish in our mind, making way for new and positive experiences... when we begin this process we are on our way not only to surviving but learning how to thrive.

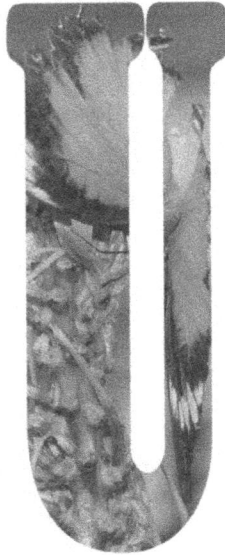

Is for...

'U' is for Understanding... Both making sense of what happened and how it has affected us and also having people around us who understand it too is crucial in healing. When we understand why we are feeling or thinking the way we do, we have the power to change it if needs be. But also sadly many people in this world fail to understand the fallout from CSA. Some because it just hasn't ever factored in their life, some because they choose to actively avoid it and some because they don't want to know and understand it through fear or maybe their own pain. A lack of understanding can cause more damage to someone who has been through CSA. Some deeply hurtful things are said through a lack of understanding. For example a relative of mine once told me that I was 'okay' now with what had happened to me! Firstly they had 'decided' for me and 'assumed' what they were saying was correct... secondly for me it showed a total lack of understanding of the agonies I have been through. Also I am sure it made them feel better about things to.

How I manage someone else's lack of understanding and reactions determines how it affects me. It is so important that we have a person or people in our lives that DO understand or at least are trying and wanting to understand. Sometimes it can feel like nobody understands our pain or our thoughts on this journey... but there are always people that will genuinely understand... we just need to find them.

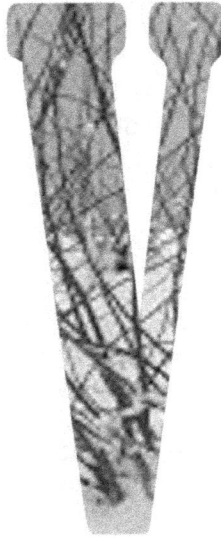

Is for...

'V' is for Valuable... So many survivors have such a low esteem about themselves (me included at times). We have endured a crime which not only steals our innocence, it strips us of feeling like a person of worth. As a result we may feel anger, hatred, self loathing. We may not place any value on who we are as a person. This in turn can send out the wrong message to others, if you do not like and respect yourself... others may feed off of the message you are sending out. Every single child born has the right to be cared for, nurtured and kept safe from harm. Survivors are no different in that, you -should- have been cared for, nurtured and kept safe from harm. The fact that something went horribly wrong in childhood says nothing about the child and everything about the wrong in our society. Yet I know from personal experience that we can blame ourselves and when I reached the point of therapy I absolutely hated my inner child. Hating my inner child in essence meant I hated my very self. For many years I didn't care if something hurt me, I felt I deserved to be hurt. The reason I didn't care was because I placed no value on who I was as a person.

I was not the prized ornament in the cabinet for 'best'... in my mind I was only fit to be taken out with the rubbish. Over a long period of time and with a lot of intervention this changed. Realising that my inner child did NOTHING wrong freed me up to like her and eventually I learnt to love her. Once I valued her things began to switch around and it was my lack of self care that went out for the rubbish! You are a person of great value & worth.

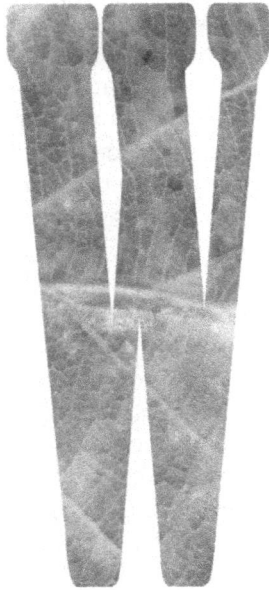

Is for...

'W' is for Warmth... In my teens and throughout my twenties as I struggled to cope with the fallout from my childhood I felt like I was in an emotional wilderness. I found myself in that place for days and months on end. It was dark, lonely and cold in that place which I couldn't seem to see a way out of. Some of that wilderness was about being so isolated from people who would have understood me. I lived in a house where nobody discussed emotions. I lived in a house where the family dynamic was so un-balanced. I spent hours and hours just shut away in my room as I felt like no one understood. I didn't have access to the internet and although I searched in the library, the books on CSA were few and mostly very wordy professional studies. If you feel like you are in the wilderness and alone... come in from the cold. Find people who understand your situation and can support you. I now know there are lots of places (mostly online) where you can find the warmth of other survivors.

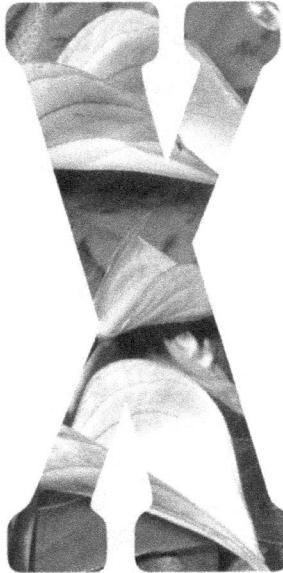

Is for...

'X' is for Xenocryst... A Xenocryst is a crystal which is foreign to the rock in which it was formed in. Many times in my life I have felt like a Xenocryst within my family. Many times I have felt like I didn't fit it and many times I did not want to fit in. My family has been at times very toxic and I had to work hard in therapy to understand my family dynamic. When you understand the games people can play (intentionally or unintentionally) then you can opt out of being caught up in them. I am glad that I have a connection to them... like the crystal was formed in a rock. However I have had to spend a long time chipping away at some of that rock to be able to be myself. To be able to find the crystal... to learn to like who I am. To understand that they are my family and I love them but I am my own person too. For the crystal to shine, it needs to be brought out into the light. Sometimes we are born into family dynamics which leave us with little esteem or confidence when faced with the world outside. Sometimes we have to chip away at the rock whatever it may be... you are a crystal and no matter what you were born into... you deserve to shine.

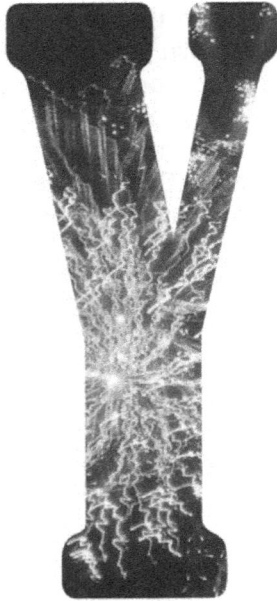

Is for...

'Y' is if You... Survivors need and deserve the right kind of help and support to begin to recover. However ultimately the healing journey belongs to YOU! It rests within your hands and it is your determination that will move you forwards. You can choose to stay where you are for many reasons. Sometimes familiarity even when it is far from ideal is less scary than the unknown... and therefore we may choose to stay in our discomfort. You may feel and rightly so that someone stole away your childhood or a part of it... however your future is there for you to take a hold of. You can spend a lot of energy on misery about the past or you can decide to use that energy to heal and invest in your future. The road to healing is tough and it takes courage to stay on the road. Nobody can do that healing work for you... nobody can live your life for you. Why not decide to be the best YOU that you can be... you owe it to yourself and all those who love and care about you.

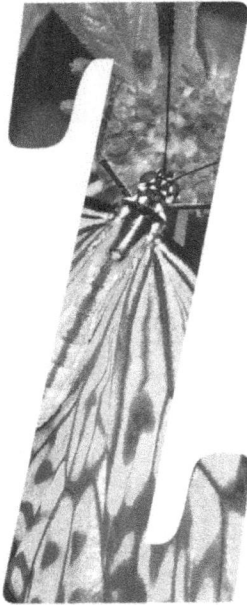

Is for...

'Z' is for Zigzag... The road called 'Healing' is not an easy one to travel. It takes so much courage and strength to face what happened to us head on. I remember on many occasions wishing that I could close the lid on the box marked 'Agonisingly painful'. The contents of that box were all the things I had buried, all the things that felt too difficult to keep remembering. Yet on the road called healing we have to take the lid off of that box and work our way through the contents. This can only be done when the time is right and you have the appropriate help you need. Along the way there may be many hiccups or moments when you feel like you can't/don't want to continue the journey. Perhaps you will take a wrong turning or get lost along the way... far from being straight this road is full of zigzags. So long as you keep on trying and you keep on returning to your healing path... the zigzags in the road won't stop you. Every day that we are here is the perfect day to start over again... every new day is waiting for you... live it well.

Kate Swift

www.ingramcontent.com/pod-product-compliance
Lightning Source LLC
Chambersburg PA
CBHW031221290326
41931CB00035B/654